I0122676

TIGHTEN YOUR BELT

OVERCOME
OBESITY

Gastric Band Surgery: A newer, safer, surgical
option that will not only help you lose weight,
but also keep it off!

DR. DUC C. VUONG

TIGHTEN
YOUR BELT

OVERCOME
OBESITY

By Dr. Duc C. Vuong

© 2008 Dr. Duc C. Vuong. All rights reserved.
The Lap-Band® is a registerd trademark of Allergan, Inc.

ISBN: 9780981454597
Library of Congress Control Number: 2008941722

Published by Escalation Press
Cover and Interior Design by Nathan Brown,
Writers of the Round Table Inc.

No part of this publication may be reproduced or transmitted in any form or by any means, mechanical or electronic, including photocopying and recording, or by any information storage and retrieval system, without permission in writing from author or publisher (except by a reviewer, who may quote brief passages and/or show brief video clips in a review).

CONTENTS

Chapter One
The Difficulty of Weight Loss

The New Health Crisis

The way we think in medicine about obesity has changed significantly over the last five years. In this new millennium, obesity is the United States' biggest health problem. Back in the eighties, it was smoking. The surgeon general required health warnings on tobacco labels, and now everyone knows that smoking is bad for you, even if some people continue to smoke. In the nineties, the health challenge was AIDS. We were all worried about different ways of contracting AIDS and HIV and how they could be treated.

Moving forward in this decade, our primary challenge is obesity. Of course, there are still significant challenges with smoking and AIDS, and the number one cause of preventable death is still smoking. But the rate of increase in smoking has slowed, and the rate of increase in obesity has climbed, making obesity the number two cause of preventable death in the U.S. I think in the next five to ten years, those numbers will switch places.

Now it is generally accepted that at least half of Americans are overweight and a third of Americans are obese. A recent news story said that by 2040, 100% of Americans will be overweight. This number seems impossible at first. Yet some studies say that already two-thirds of Americans are overweight, so we are almost there.

Obesity is a serious health concern because it increases our morbidity, meaning we have more illnesses. It also increases our mortality, or risk of death. Depending on what study you read, obesity costs our country up to $200 BILLION per year in illnesses and health-related costs. This number increases every year as more Americans move from normal weight to overweight status and from overweight to obese categories.

The number I like to point out is that every year, our nation spends $33 billion dollars on weight-loss products: Weight-Watchers, SlimFast, Jenny Craig, Nutrisystem, Atkins, Zone, South Beach, Herbalife, Alli, even products made from snail shells advertised on late-night television. There are too many weight-loss products and companies to mention here, and more appear on the market all the time. This huge industry, as is indicated by the rapidly rising rates of obesity, is not making our country thinner and healthier. It is not educating our nation on how to make smarter choices. Its goal is to make money. By keeping consumers dependent on their products, they buy more and company profits rise. If people could make healthy choices on their own, they would not need to spend money on these products. Therefore, it is not in the best interest of these companies to educate the American public or, in fact, to provide long-term weight-loss solutions.

As a doctor and a father, I am very concerned about the growing rates of obesity. I ultimately want my patients to be smart. Even if you decide that surgery is not the right option for you, at least after reading this book you will know some tips and be able to make better decisions on your own. Health is one of the most important things in the world. Without it, nothing else matters much. It is important that we all understand how the choices we make impact our health and know how we can improve our health to lead more fulfilling lives.

What does obese mean and how is obesity changing our country?

You cannot determine if your weight is healthy just by the number on the scale. Two-hundred and fifty pounds is very different for someone who is five feet tall and someone who is six feet tall. Doctors use something called the Body Mass Index (BMI), which is a formula factoring in both weight and height. The formula is a little cumbersome to perform, so most doctors provide patients with a chart, similar to the one below.

A healthy BMI is under 25, overweight is 25-30, obese is 30-35, severely obese is 35-40, and morbidly obese is over 40. We have a new term now for BMI's over 50 called super-obese. This is the category you see on reality TV shows like *Big Medicine*.

Body Mass Index Table

	Normal						Overweight					Obese									
BMI	19	20	21	22	23	24	25	26	27	28	29	30	31	32	33	34	35	36	37	38	39
Height (inches)																		Body Weight (pounds)			
58	91	96	100	105	110	115	119	124	129	134	138	143	148	153	158	162	167	172	177	181	186
59	94	99	104	109	114	119	124	128	133	138	143	148	153	158	163	168	173	178	183	188	193
60	97	102	107	112	118	123	128	133	138	143	148	153	158	163	168	174	179	184	189	194	199
61	100	106	111	116	122	127	132	137	143	148	153	158	164	169	174	180	185	190	195	201	206
62	104	109	115	120	126	131	136	142	147	153	158	164	169	175	180	186	191	196	202	207	213
63	107	113	118	124	130	135	141	146	152	158	163	169	175	180	186	191	197	203	208	214	220
64	110	116	122	128	134	140	145	151	157	163	169	174	180	186	192	197	204	209	215	221	227
65	114	120	126	132	138	144	150	156	162	168	174	180	186	192	198	204	210	216	222	228	234
66	118	124	130	136	142	148	155	161	167	173	179	186	192	198	204	210	216	223	229	235	241
67	121	127	134	140	146	153	159	166	172	178	185	191	198	204	211	217	223	230	236	242	249
68	125	131	138	144	151	158	164	171	177	184	190	197	203	210	216	223	230	236	243	249	256
69	128	135	142	149	155	162	169	176	182	189	196	203	209	216	223	230	236	243	250	257	263
70	132	139	146	153	160	167	174	181	188	195	202	209	216	222	229	236	243	250	257	264	271
71	136	143	150	157	165	172	179	186	193	200	208	215	222	229	236	243	250	257	265	272	279
72	140	147	154	162	169	177	184	191	199	206	213	221	228	235	242	250	258	265	272	279	287
73	144	151	159	166	174	182	189	197	204	212	219	227	235	242	250	257	265	272	280	288	295
74	148	155	163	171	179	186	194	202	210	218	225	233	241	249	256	264	272	280	287	295	303
75	152	160	168	176	184	192	200	208	216	224	232	240	248	256	264	272	279	287	295	303	311
76	156	164	172	180	189	197	205	213	221	230	238	246	254	263	271	279	287	295	304	312	320

Source: Adapted from *Clinical Guidelines on the Identification, Evaluation, and Treatment of Overweight and Obesity in Adults: The Evidence Report*.

In 1985 the Center for Disease Control (CDC) realized they needed to figure out what was happening with body weight in this country. They began collecting data across states, but there were many with no data.. We don't really have complete statistics until 1995. In the 1995 figure below, the dark states have 15-19% of their population with a BMI of 30 or more (remember, a BMI of 30 or more is obese). But by 2006, the last year for which we have data, there are no states except for Hawaii with obesity rates under 15%, and the light-colored states have pretty much disappeared. Most of the country has moved into

Body Mass Index

Used as indicator of excess body fat
Body Mass Index (BMI) = Weight(kg)/Height(m)2

NORMAL BMI 18.5 - 24.9	OVERWEIGHT BMI 25 - 29.9	OBESE BMI 30-34.9	SEVERELY OBESE BMI 35-39.9	MORBIDLY OBESE BMI ≥ 40

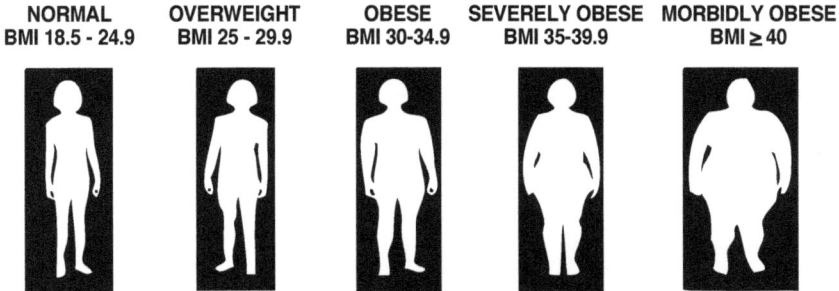

obesity rates that did not exist for any state a decade earlier. And this is with the United States public spending $33 billion per year on weight-loss products. This approach to weight loss clearly does not work.

The obesity problem in our children is especially disturbing and is reaching epidemic proportions. A recent cover story in *Newsweek* addressed rising obesity rates among American children, and more magazine and television stories are covering this worrisome topic. We have started our overweight kids on blood pressure medicines, diabetes medicines that are intended for adults, and cholesterol medicines that are known to be harmful to adult livers, much less adolescent livers. Furthermore, there is solid scientific evidence that shows that if overweight teenagers become overweight young adults, it is highly probable that they will remain overweight for the rest of their lives. It becomes too hard for them to lose weight because their behaviors have become ingrained. Everyone loves Jerry from Subway, but he is a very rare exception to this trend.

Obesity Trends* Among U.S. Adults
BRFSS, 1995
(*BMI ≥ 30, or ~ 30lbs overweight for 5'4" person)

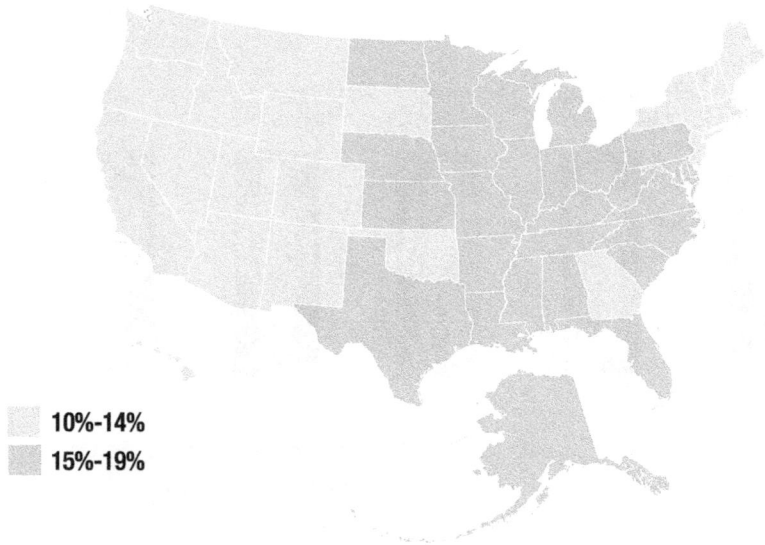

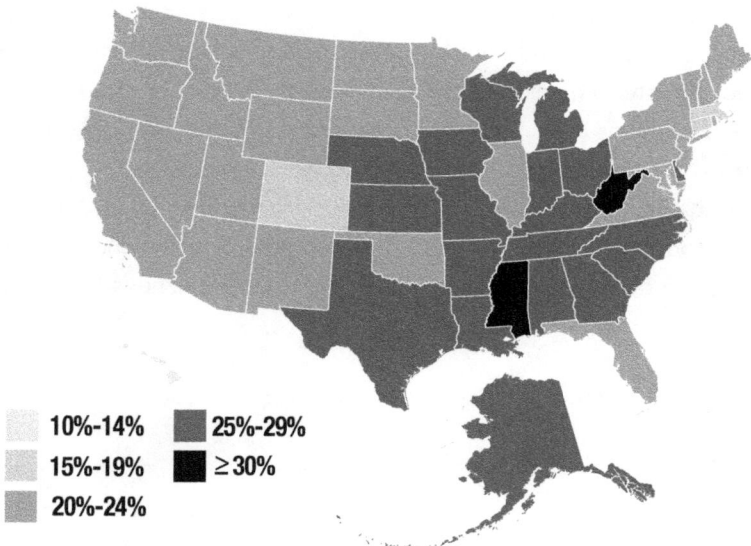

▨	**10%-14%**
▨	**15%-19%**

Obesity Trends Among U.S. Adults
BRFSS, 2006
(*BMI ≥ 30, or ~ 30lbs overweight for 5'4" person)

▨	**10%-14%**	▨	**25%-29%**
▨	**15%-19%**	■	**≥ 30%**
▨	**20%-24%**		

Obesity:

The percentage of the population older than 15 with a body-mass index greater than 30.

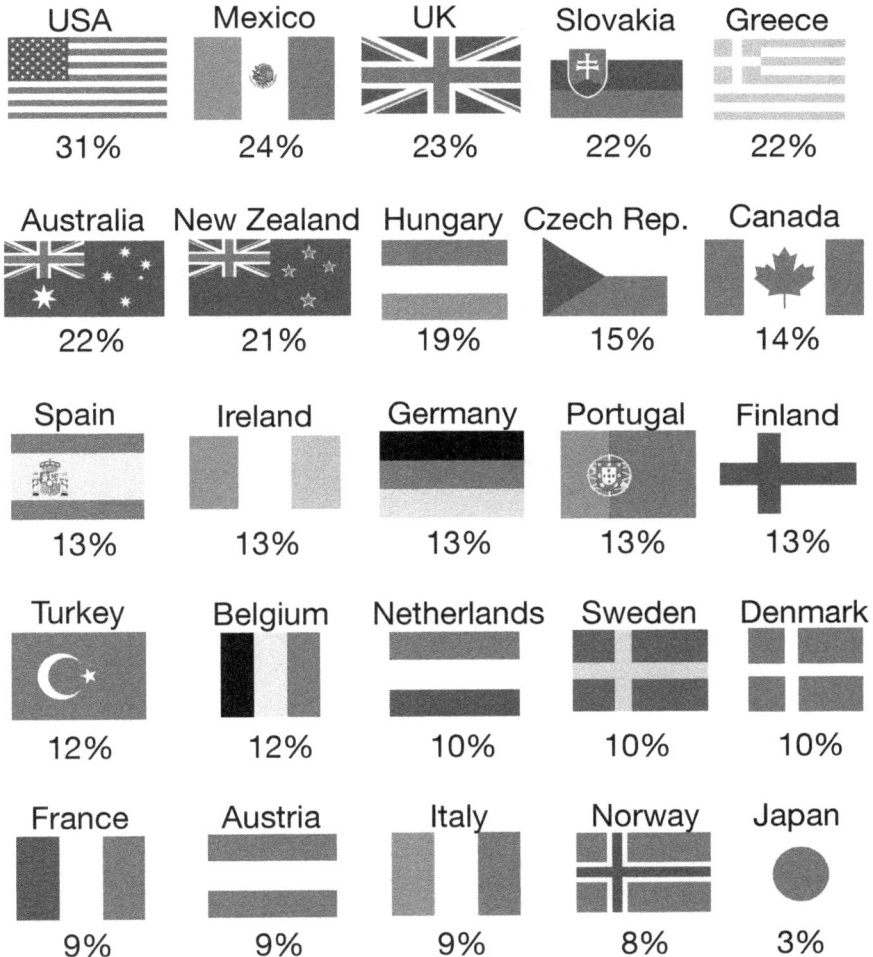

USA	Mexico	UK	Slovakia	Greece
31%	24%	23%	22%	22%

Australia	New Zealand	Hungary	Czech Rep.	Canada
22%	21%	19%	15%	14%

Spain	Ireland	Germany	Portugal	Finland
13%	13%	13%	13%	13%

Turkey	Belgium	Netherlands	Sweden	Denmark
12%	12%	10%	10%	10%

France	Austria	Italy	Norway	Japan
9%	9%	9%	8%	3%

The United States leads the world in obesity. Thirty-one percent of Americans are obese. The runners-up are our neighbors in Mexico, with obesity rates of 24%, and the United Kingdom at 23%. The Austrians, French, and Italians have only 9% obesity in their populations. The Japanese and Koreans trail at only three percent. So we are truly world leaders—in obesity rates.

The hated E-word

Food is one part of the weight equation. We have a vast selection of fast, convenient, calorie-dense food. Unfortunately, the stuff that is the worst for you is also very cheap and available at nearly every corner. At Taco Bell, you can have a big meal for three dollars.

Exercise is the other part of the equation. Not only are we eating more every day, we are moving around less. We are simply not expending all those extra calories we consume. I'm not referring to going out for a jog or lifting weights – I'm referring to the small movements that comprise every day activities. For example, we never get up to change the TV channel any more, and we get our food, money, and prescriptions while waiting in our cars. Everything is so convenient now, and we grow accustomed to that. I'll spend half an hour trying to find the remote control so I don't have to turn the TV on myself. It may not seem like much, but these small changes in our daily activity levels add up and can lead to significant weight gain.

	Here is a picture of an old push mower. When I was a kid, we would see them all the time.
	Then people started to get riding mowers so they wouldn't have to walk back and forth across their lawns and fight with the starter cord.
	Have you seen this? It is the lawnmower of the future. It is virtually a robot that mows up to one acre on a single charge, and all you have to do is sit back and watch it. It certainly makes the little push mower seem archaic.

There are vacuum cleaners along these lines as well that scoot across the floor on their own and track down the dirt and scare the pets all by themselves. Adding up the energy we used to spend pushing the lawn mower, climbing the stairs, walking our dogs, bicycling to the corner store, running to catch the bus to work, and even standing up to change the channel, our less convenient, older way of life amounted to a lot more calories expended on a daily basis without doing any special exercise.

I give my patients a pedometer so they can track how much they walk each day and try to increase their activity. Many physicians and health experts recommend walking 10,000 steps throughout the day. It is difficult to walk this amount every day; unless you have a physically demanding profession or make it a point to exercise, it is likely that you walk about half the recommended amount or even less. Our lifestyles have become very comfortable and very free of the need to move around.

Why we need to change the trend

There are numerous comorbidities of being overweight. Diabetes, high blood pressure, high cholesterol, joint disease, asthma, reflux, and sleep apnea are ones many people have heard of or experienced. But did you know that cancer is linked to being overweight? We have solid research now that correlates being overweight with higher incidence of certain types of cancer. For example, there is a strong correlation between obesity and breast cancer. Typically women who are overweight have more breast tissue, and having more breast tissue is a key risk factor for breast cancer. Also, overweight women are exposed to higher levels of estrogen, which is also related to breast cancer. There is a direct correlation between obesity and colon cancer as well. If you are eating fast foods and highly processed foods, you will likely be overweight and will not have the good colon health that comes from eating fresh vegetables and whole grains. There is also a strong correlation between obesity and uterine cancer, endometrial cancer, and stomach cancers.

Another side effect of obesity is infertility. Do you know anyone who is trying to get pregnant and spends $17,000 or so on endometrial fertilization? Many weight-loss patients who were spending fortunes on fertility treatments would lose around 25 pounds and get pregnant right away.

Studies have shown that with a BMI of just thirty, which is borderline between overweight and obese, people have a 55% increase in mortality (death), a 70% increase in coronary heart disease (heart attack), a 75% increase in stroke, and a 400% increase in diabetes. Four hundred percent! (I will share some good news about diabetes in a little bit.)

If you are a man between the ages of twenty-five and thirty-five and have a BMI of 30, you have twelve times the chances of dying as a normal weight man. You have only a 33% chance of living to the age of 65 – and sixty-five is not considered old anymore! We meet eighty-five and ninety year-old people all the time now. The last time sixty-five was considered old was when Roosevelt was figuring out social security. The average lifespan then was sixty-seven, so the administration wanted to establish social security benefits to start at sixty-five. The long life spans we have now are wonderful, even if they are contributing to the social security crisis. Sadly, the average American life expectancy in 2007 decreased for the first time ever, and this decrease is because of higher rates of obesity and the corresponding comorbidities.

It gets worse the heavier you are, and it is not a direct relationship. It is exponential, a ski slope! By the time your BMI is forty, your relative risk of dying is three times as high as someone who is normal weight.

Body Mass Index vs. Mortality
Exponential Increase in Risk

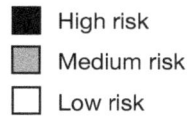

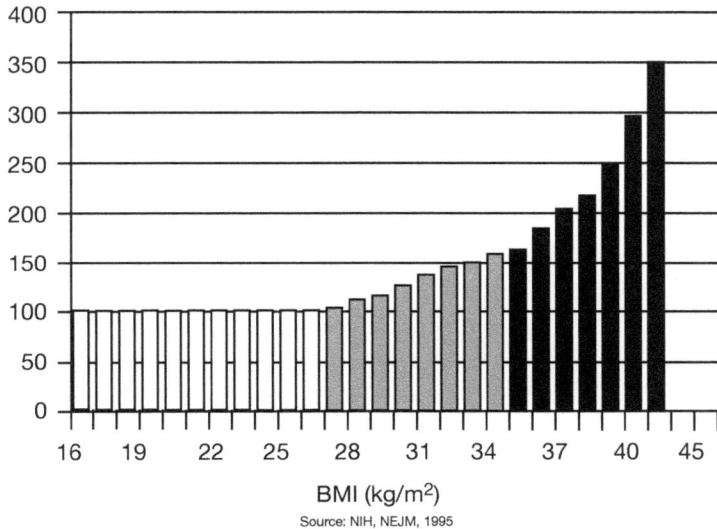

■ High risk
▨ Medium risk
☐ Low risk

BMI (kg/m^2)

Source: NIH, NEJM, 1995

The costs of treating the obese, diabetic, and hypertensive patient with medicine is over $1000 every month in many cases. A fairly typical array of medicines includes insulin, syringes, and testing strips for diabetes; two medications for blood pressure; a reflux pill; a medication for cholesterol; another drug or two for arthritis; and often something for depression. Many overweight patients are prescribed an antidepressant because they tell their doctor that they are tired all the time, do not have energy any more, or do not want to do things they used to enjoy doing. These are the exact symptoms of depression, even though the patient may feel this way because of arthritis and exhaustion.

In one month, these medications add up to $1100. In one year, that's almost $14,000 just for one person's medicines. You could have bought two of those fancy lawn mowers for this amount! And this number does not reflect when you feel bad and miss work or otherwise lose potential income.

Notes

Notes

Chapter Two
Surgical Solutions

Now for some good news

The first time I saw this chart, I thought that it indicated more bad news about obesity – I thought it meant that 95% of overweight patients have diabetes and 75% have sleep apnea.

Comorbidity Improvement with Weight Loss

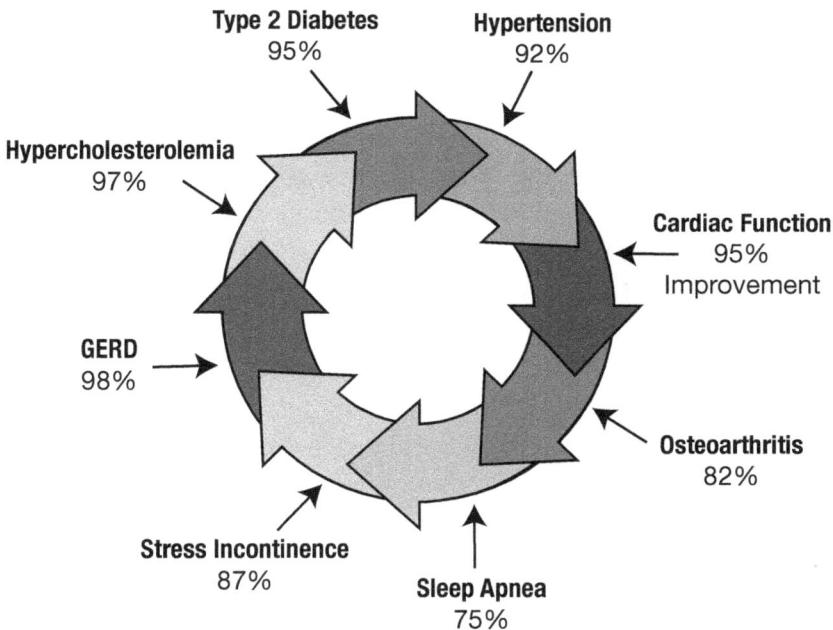

Type 2 Diabetes
95%

Hypertension
92%

Hypercholesterolemia
97%

Cardiac Function
95%
Improvement

GERD
98%

Osteoarthritis
82%

Stress Incontinence
87%

Sleep Apnea
75%

But this diagram actually shows the percentage of patients whose illnesses improve when they lose excess weight. We can see some impressive numbers here: 95% of overweight patients who lose weight will have improvement in their diabetes, 75% will have improvement in sleep apnea. Even more impressively, about 73% will be *cured* of their diabetes – not just treated with another pill or another shot but actually cured. 98% will have improvement in Gastroesophogeal Reflux Disease (GERD). So far, 100% of my patients have been cured of their reflux, and that alone made it worthwhile to them to lose weight.

The following comes from an article that came out in 2007 in the *New England Journal of Medicine,* one of the most respected medical publications in the world. The article describes a landmark study, which means a study that follows a large number of patients for many years. This particular study followed nearly 8000 people who dieted and exercised (the control group) and 8000 people who had the open gastric bypass surgery (which was the only surgical option back when the study started). Doctors followed the health of these people for an average of about seven years, and occasionally as long as ten years.

They found that those with the open gastric bypass surgery who had lost weight reduced their chance of dying by 40%. At first, 40% does not sound so impressive, but if this were a cancer drug study and there was even a 20% difference in survival rates, everybody would be on that new drug! 40% is a huge number when someone's life is at stake. In addition, the study indicates that the surgical patients' chances of dying from a heart attack decreased by 56%, their chances of dying from complications of diabetes decreased by 92%, and their risk of dying from cancer decreased by 60%.

This is a study that has changed many doctors' opinions about how to treat their overweight patients, but not all doctors are aware of it. You may want to look up this article, read it on your own, and ask your doctor about it.

Isn't surgery risky?

Many people focus on the risks of weight-loss surgery, and they are certainly something to consider. However, the risks should not mean that surgery is a last resort, as it has been regarded historically. According to recent research, your chances of dying if you are obese are far worse if you do not do anything about your weight than if you undergo a weight-loss procedure. After one year of the *New England* study, the two groups of people, those who continued to try to diet and exercise and those who had the open gastric bypass surgery, had the same death rates. After seven years, those who did not have the surgery had much higher death rates. This means that in the short-term the risks of doing nothing and having the surgery are the same, and that in the long-term it is far riskier to remain overweight than to have the surgery.

Doctors and patients are starting to change their thinking about surgery. Some surgeries were risky back in the 1970s and even 1980s. But times have changed and there are now surgical options that are far safer than the open gastric bypass surgery that was the focus of this study. With the newer and safer surgical options, the death rates from weight-loss surgery are even lower.

What should I look for in a surgeon?

In 1991 the National Institute of Health (NIH) started to give doctors some guidelines on when we should and whom we should operate on. Honestly, these guidelines are primarily for insurance purposes, but most doctors will adhere to them. Here are the criteria a patient and surgeon must meet according to these guidelines:

1. NIH (and your insurance company) want the patient to have a BMI of over 40 or a BMI of 35 with one or two comorbidities, like high blood pressure, diabetes, or arthritis. Depending on your insurance company, sleep apnea will usually count as a comorbidity, too.

2. The surgeon must provide a clinical environment supporting all aspects of management and assessment. That means the surgeon needs to prepare you as well as possible for surgery: talk with your doctors, control your blood pressure, control your diabetes, and basically make it safe for you to have surgery. Once the surgeon does the surgery and you lose weight, there needs to be a procedure to adjust your medicines appropriately. This procedure requires careful communication with your other doctors.

3. After surgery, lifelong medical surveillance of the patient is necessary. To me, this is absolutely essential, yet it is the aspect most commonly overlooked by surgeons and patients. In establishing this as a criterion for insurance coverage, NIH recognized that surgery is a tool, not a magic bullet. It amazes me how many surgical weight-loss programs are out there that provide very little post-surgery support. And in my opinion, these programs will not be effective in the long-run.

This last criterion indicates a paradigm shift in our understanding of obesity, even if it has not changed the thinking of all surgeons yet. We now think of obesity as a chronic disease. In America, it is too hard to lose weight and maintain weight loss for it to be understood as a temporary condition. Obesity is a chronic illness just like diabetes, just like high blood pressure, and just like AIDS. With the lifelong medical surveillance requirement from NIH, it is not enough for a surgeon to slap a Lap-Band around you and send you to your family reunion to see who can eat the most ribs. That's no way to be successful. A surgical program has to take into consideration your entire life and help you make changes that will allow you to be successful with your new surgical tool. That does not happen overnight or automatically after the surgery.

I think the surgeon you choose is not nearly as important as the program his or her clinic provides. The Lap-Band surgery is fairly straightforward and you do not need a highly skilled and specialized surgeon to have it safely and effectively performed. You do need an environment that will help you adapt to life with the Lap-Band and help you develop strategies to face challenges throughout your life that could sabotage your weight loss.

Remember: It's not the surgeon but the program that is most important for long-term weight-loss success.

What can I expect from weight-loss surgery?

There have been a lot of weight-loss surgeries developed throughout the years, so patients have choices. The surgeries work through different mechanisms: some work through restricting how much you can eat, while some work through malabsorption. Some work very quickly, some are slow and steady. Some are really risky, some are quite safe. The two surgical options that have really stood the test of time are the Lap-Band and the Roux-en-Y bypass, also known as gastric bypass.

With all these different options, we have to keep in mind that surgery is really not an easy way out. It is meant to be a tool that you need to learn how to use most effectively, and so it is wise to be part of a clinical setting or practice that is interested in helping you change your behaviors. It is very hard to do it by yourself. Nearly everyone has tried diet and exercise on their own before, and it may work for a while. But changing long-standing behaviors is hard to sustain without a support network.

The goal of surgery, whatever kind you choose, is to improve your health and your quality of life. The surgery may well lengthen your life span and increase your active enjoyment of life. For me, both of these aspects are important; your doctor should aim to help you become healthier and enjoy a healthier lifestyle. If you are constantly worrying about food and exercise, you might not enjoy your newfound health. A good program can help you find a happy balance.

Remember that while you may end up feeling more attractive after you lose excess weight, weight-loss surgery is not a cosmetic procedure. Cosmetic improvement may be a side effect, but it is just that. You will not wake up looking like a supermodel. Remember that even with surgery, weight loss takes time.

The first surgical option: Gastric Bypass

Patients have decisions to make after they decide to have weight loss surgery. Gastric bypass or Lap-Band is a first decision.

Many of my patients know people who have had the gastric bypass. They are often impressed with their friends' rapid weight loss, but then notice these people are sick a lot of the time, have poor nutrition, or return to their previous weight after a while. These side effects result from the nature of the surgery itself.

In gastric bypass surgery, the surgeon staples off a little pouch about the size of a walnut formed out of the top portion of the patient's stomach. He or she then disconnects the end of the intestines, moves it up, and reconnects it up top.

Postoperative Anatomy of the Gastric Bypass

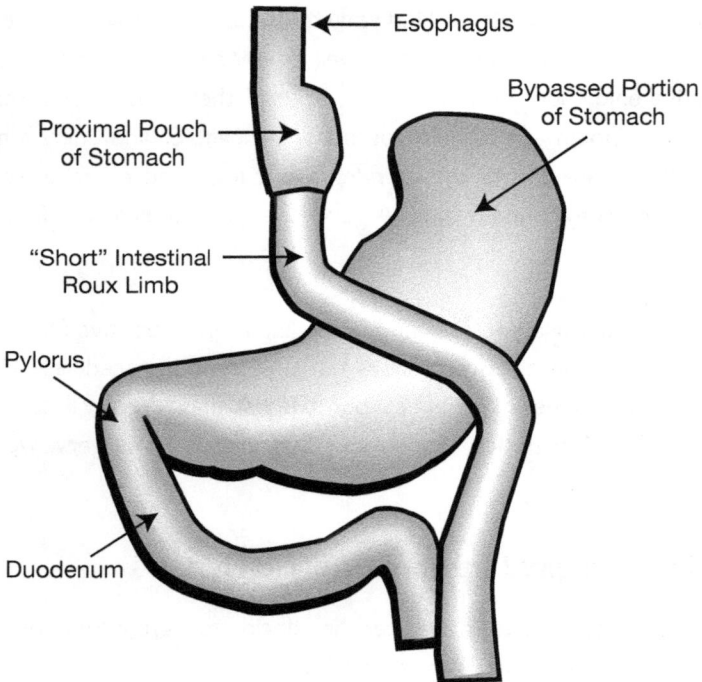

This means that the lower part of the stomach and the upper part of the intestines are no longer involved in eating and digestion. When the patient eats, the food sits in the little pouch, passes through and combines with the digestive stomach juices. It causes weight loss for two reasons: the stomach area is smaller, so the patient feels full on far less food, and the upper intestines are bypassed, meaning that less of the food is absorbed.

Gastric bypass is an effective surgery, and patients may lose up to 80% of their excess weight in the first year after the surgery. By excess weight, we mean that if you are 100 pounds overweight you would lose 80 pounds. This is the percentage we care about, not your total weight lost. This is for the same reason we use the BMI chart: 80 pounds may be a huge amount on a five-foot tall woman and only a moderate amount on a six-foot-four man. Most people keep the weight off for quite a while and most people will have improvements in their illnesses.

But gastric bypass surgery comes with some complications. One is called dumping syndrome. If patients eat too much refined sugar, it causes bad diarrhea, lightheadedness, and possibly fainting spells. Sometimes the surgery works too well and patients lose weight so quickly they become malnourished. You can tell because their hair might be brittle, their skin might look grey, and they might act lethargic. Because part of the intestine is bypassed, fewer nutrients are absorbed from the food, which might result in osteoporosis, vitamin deficiencies, and anemia.

Also, the operative death rate on average is about 1-2%. A good surgeon would still have a 1% death rate – that is one patient out of 100! This rate is too high for me to feel comfortable with this type of surgery.

I have also had to operate on patients who had internal complications from the surgery. My first year as a surgeon, I took care of three patients who had internal twisting of their intestines where they were reconnected. I had to operate on them in the middle of the night because they had dangerous leakage, and they were sick in the hospital for two to four weeks.

Also, it is possible for a patient, especially one who has not been well educated on nutrition and does not change his or her eating habits, to stretch out the stomach pouch. After a couple of years of continued poor eating habits, it is possible for the stomach pouch to contain as much as their pre-operative whole stomach could. The patient will then feel hungry more often and be able to eat larger amounts of food. This is why many gastric bypass patients regain their weight a few years after surgery.

Hernias, blood clots, hair loss, gallstones, and a host of other problems also pose long-term risks to gastric bypass patients.

The newer, safer surgical option: the Lap-Band

The ideal weight-loss surgery is the one that is safest and most effective. A safer surgery is usually the least invasive and disrupts the way the body is naturally made as little as possible. An effective surgery should not merely allow for weight-loss immediately afterwards but also keep the patient at a lower weight over time. Nearly everyone I talk to who is looking into bariatric (weight-loss) surgery has at some point lost weight, but then they have put it all back on plus more. Losing weight is the easy part of the battle, because keeping it off is very hard indeed.

Keep in mind that there is no perfect surgery, but the side effects should be minimal. A good surgery also needs to be reproducible, meaning that nearly any well-trained surgeon should be able to do the surgery. It is not practical if a patient has to travel far to find the one person who can safely perform the surgery. An effective weight-loss surgery also needs to be adjustable so you can control how quickly or slowly patients lose weight.

Finally, the ideal surgery would be reversible so that if a patient does not like it or encounters reasons that render it impractical, it can be undone. Gastric bypass doctors often say the surgery is reversible. It is, but it is very hard to perform the surgery that would reverse it, much harder than performing the gastric bypass in the first place.

You should consider whether you want a surgeon who does an open surgery, which is traditional, or a laproscopic surgery, which uses tiny cameras and very small incisions. Laproscopic surgery is popular for gall bladder removal and a variety of other procedures, including scar tissue removal. It is usually much safer for the patient, because it requires smaller incisions, and patients usually heal faster afterwards.

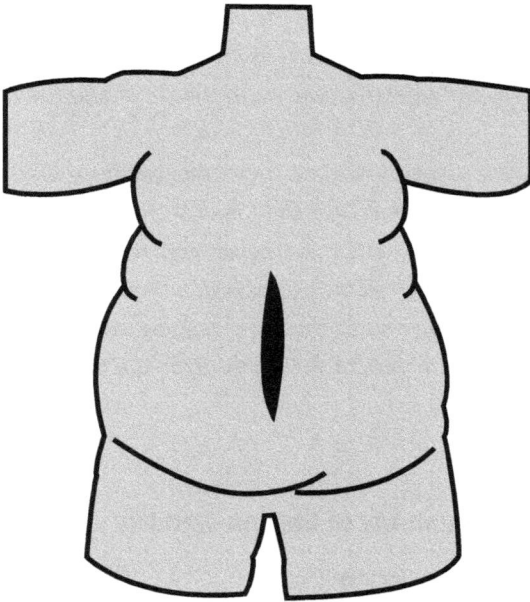

The incision location, number of incisions and the incision size vary from sugeon to surgeon.

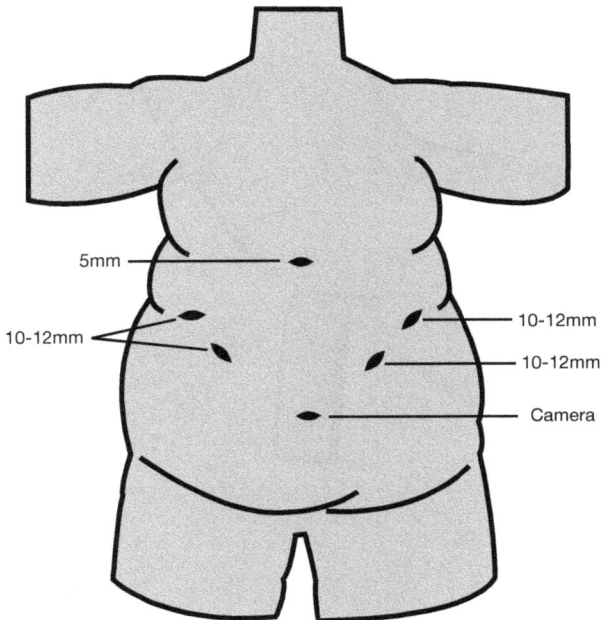

The best surgical choice for me and for my patients is laparoscopic adjustable gastric banding, most commonly known as the Lap-Band. It is simple, safe, completely reversible, and effective over both the short and the long term.

During the surgery, the surgeon will first move the liver to the side so it is not injured during the surgery, then slide the Lap-Band around the top part of the stomach. The Lap-Band is a silicone device much like a belt with its own buckle that wraps around the stomach, making a little pouch about the size of a walnut. To decrease the risk of the band slipping down the stomach, the surgeon will sew the bottom part of the stomach to the top pouch.

Postoperative Anatomy of the Lap-Band®

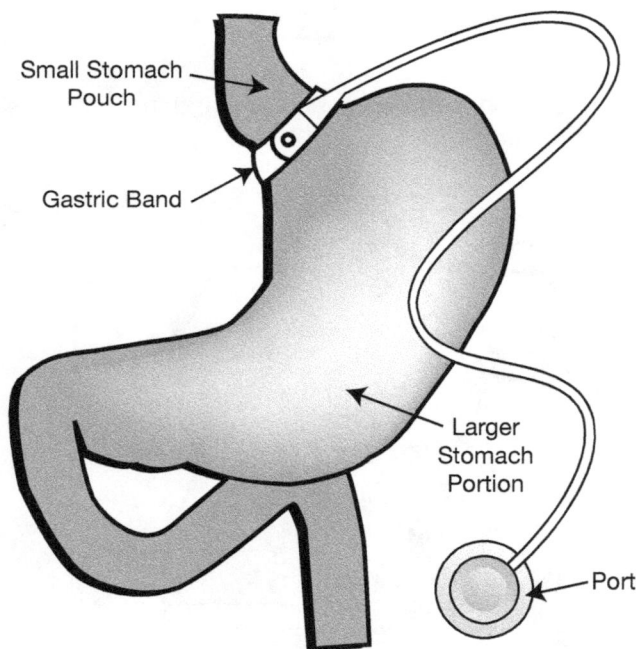

Unlike with gastric bypass, nothing is cut – there are just a couple of stitches added. Most surgeons always put three stitches on top and one on the bottom. That way, if a surgeon needs to remove the Band, it will be clear exactly how many stitches need to be removed.

The Lap-Band® Tool
FDA Aprroved in 2001

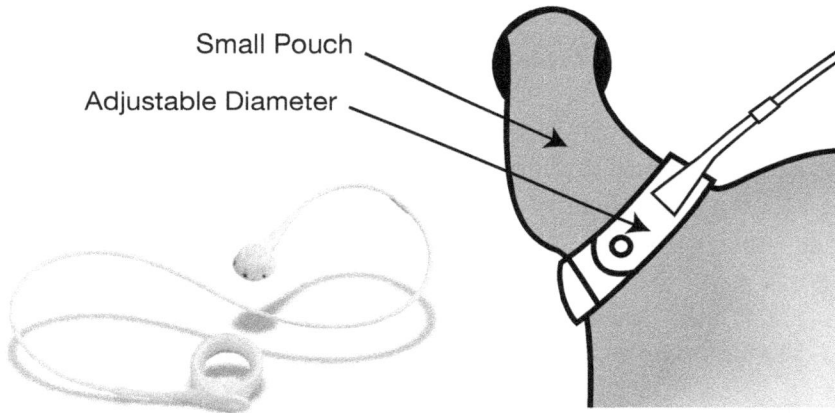

Small Pouch

Adjustable Diameter

As part of the Lap-Band surgery, the surgeon will include a port that stays underneath your skin. You will not see the port, but might be able to feel it. This is accessed with a needle (it does not hurt) that inflates the balloon around the band with fluid, creating a squeezing mechanism that controls the rate of weight loss. If the balloon is inflated too much, no food can get through. Then we just take out a little fluid and the patient can eat some food comfortably. The food sits in the little pouch and as it is digested, it slowly passes down.

The surgery itself is typically out-patient. Most of my patients have gone home the same day. Remember that you will need to have another responsible adult with you on the day of your surgery, even if you take a taxi. I send my patients to surgery in a limousine because I want them to feel pampered, like this is a fabulous start to their new lives.

Lap-Band surgery was FDA approved in the United States in 2001. This is important to keep in mind when evaluating the effectiveness of weight-loss surgeries your colleagues or family may have had. When word got out that I was going to start doing Lap-Band surgeries, a woman approached me and said she had the Lap-Band, but it did not work. When I asked when she had it done, she said 1995. Since she had the surgery done in the United States, this was not the Lap-Band! So if someone says they had the Lap-Band surgery and it did not work, ask when it was done. If it was before 2001, they probably had the Vertical Banded Gastroplasty (VBG). There is a band in there, but it is not the Lap-Band and it is not adjustable.

Another important date is June 2007, when the Lap-Band was redesigned. This new version is called the AP Lap-Band. It is a little thicker and the balloon extends all the way around. This device has even fewer complications and greater effectiveness.

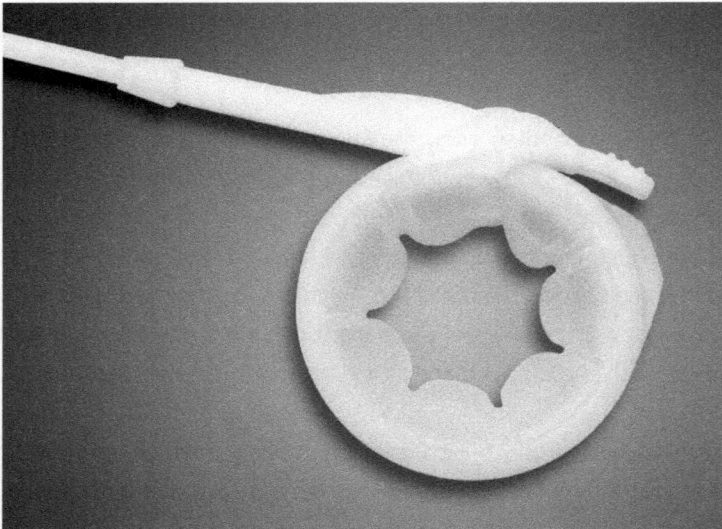

Optifast and the Lap-Band

I require my patients to follow an Optifast meal-replacement program for two weeks before surgery. Other surgeons may use different meal-replacements, and others do not require this at all. I recommend finding a surgeon who requires some meal-replacement before the surgery because it significantly shrinks the liver. The surgeon needs to reach under the liver and move it out of the way to put on the band, and you want this to be as easy as possible. When I traveled around the country observing different ways of performing Lap-Band surgery, I met plenty of doctors who did not do anything to reduce their patients' liver size. You could call a surgeon and have surgery tomorrow if you have the money and do not eat anything after midnight. But I saw doctors struggling with big livers, which increases the risk of cutting the liver and makes the band very difficult to insert, meaning that the surgery takes a longer time to perform (this increases risk of complications). With the meal-replacement plan I require, I have never had problems with the liver.

I also put patients on Optifast for a week after surgery. There is a lot of swelling around where the Lap-Band is placed after the surgery. The swelling means food could get stuck on its way to the stomach and the patient would vomit. This increases the risk of slippage, which I'll talk about in a later section. While it may seem unappealing to be on a meal-replacement program for three weeks, the benefits and increased safety make it well worth the effort.

The reason I choose to use Optifast is because it is the Cadillac of all liquid supplements. It has been around for 30 years, has been tested in multiple journals, and has proven its worth. It is also the first product to have received an ISO 9001 certification. Recently there was a pet food contamination scare across the U.S. Out of the millions of cans of pet food sold every year, all of which seem to be identical, the government narrowed the source of contamination down to one shipment that came from China. They were able to do that because of this ISO certification, which clarifies exactly what goes into every product and where it is produced. Over-the-counter weight-loss or meal-replacement products do not have this certification, so they are not regulated. Hoodia, for example, is an herb that comes from a cactus in Africa that natives of the region would eat to suppress their appetite during long treks across the desert. But last year Consumer Reports tested a bottle of Hoodia and found that 40% of the tablets in that bottle contained no cactus ingredient. You have no idea what you are taking when you buy those over-the-counter supplements. Most are a waste of money – as can be seen by the growing obesity rates that go hand-in-hand with the growing number of weight-loss products for sale. With Optifast, you know what you are getting.

Notes

Notes

Chapter Three
Life After Surgery

Life with the Lap-Band

With the Lap-Band, the patient will eat a small plate of food three times a day, will feel full, and will stay full until his or her next meal. Numerous studies have shown this. Some of my patients were skeptical that they could become full after such a small amount of food, but they do.

A Lap-Band clinic's goal is to get patients into what we call the green zone (the middle area of the diagram below). This is the point where a patient enjoyably eats and feels full after a small plate of food and stays satisfied for several hours. The green zone leads to healthy weight loss or weight maintenance.

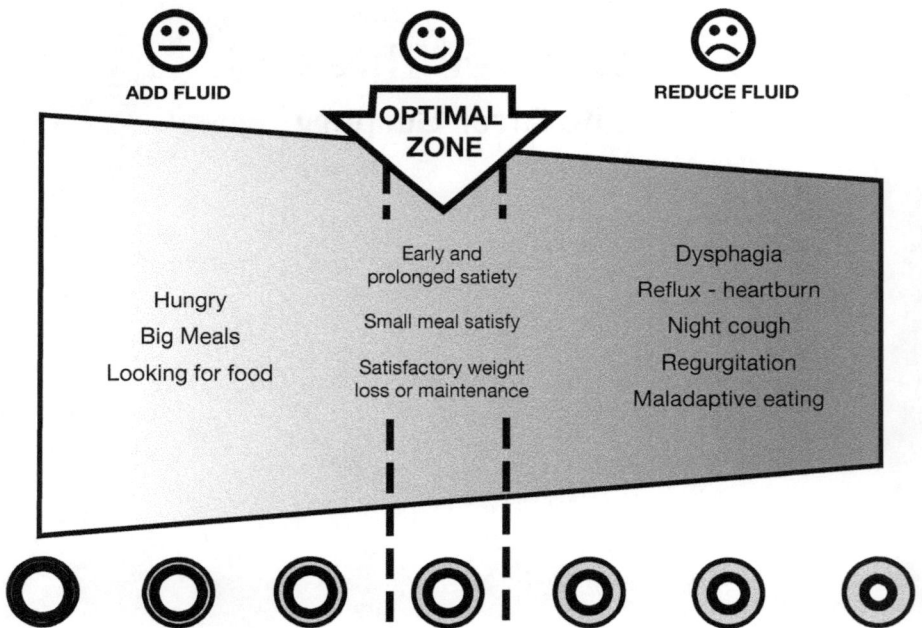

It may take a couple of adjustments to get there and other periodic adjustments to stay there over the years. The beauty of the Lap-Band is that it can be adjusted to meet the individual needs of each patient. With a good Lap-Band clinic, you will not have the problem some gastric bypass patients encounter where they lose too much weight, are malnourished, lose some hair, and look quite sickly. You also will not gain the weight back after a couple of years, as many gastric bypass patients do, since you can have periodic adjustments to make sure that you continue to stay full on small quantities of food.

If you are in the yellow zone (the left portion of the diagram), you are often hungry, eat too much, and always think about food. That means we need to add a little fluid to the band to tighten up the opening. If you have bad reflux, everything feels like it's getting stuck except for milkshakes (they are a powerful force nothing can stop!), then you are in the red zone (the right part of the diagram). The band is too tight and we need to remove a little fluid. Some patients want me to make the band really tight so that they will lose huge amounts of weight before some big event, but this is not the point of the surgery and it is not healthy. The Lap-Band should allow for you to lose weight at a moderate rate and keep it off, all while you learn to develop a healthy relationship with food. This comes with time and education.

Crunching the numbers

Here is a little quiz that I give to people who attend my seminars about the Lap-Band:

1. How many calories a day is the average person supposed to eat? Most of my prospective patients will significantly underestimate this before they start my program. They will guess 900, 1200, or 1500 calories.

    A: 2000 calories a day is the recommended daily allowance. When you read the nutrition information on the back of a food product, the percentages of recommended daily allowances are based on a 2000 calorie a day diet.

2. If you join Weight Watchers or Jenny Craig, how many calories do they have you eat a day?

Some of my prospective patients guess 1200 or so, but many have no idea. This is because the programs do not tell you. Foods are divided into categories and assigned letters, numbers, or colors. The programs do this to sell you their services and make you dependent on their coding system. If you leave their program, you gain the weight back and then join them again. They do not want you to be educated, because then you might achieve similar results on your own or with a group of friends, and they would lose the business. A good Lap-Band clinic should carefully educate you about nutrition so that you are empowered to make your own decisions. They should also be able to direct you towards books, articles, and web sites that offer helpful information about nutrition and exercise.

A: These programs bring you down to 1500 calories a day. This is also about the average for South Beach, Atkins, and other popular diets.

3.   How many calories equal one pound?

Many people also underestimate this number, guessing about 2000. They expect weight-loss from dieting and exercise to be rapid. Many diets do appear to help you lose weight rapidly, but often you are merely losing water weight at first because you are consuming less sodium. The ten pounds you might shed during your first week on some diet plans are not comprised of fat.

A: 3500 calories equals one pound. So if I regularly eat the recommended 2000 calories a day and join a program that has me eat 1500 calories a day, I create a deficit of 500 calories a day. After seven days, the deficit is 3500 calories. So the various weight-loss programs tell you to expect to lose one pound a week. Sound familiar?

If you have a well-adjusted Lap-Band and can eat three meals a day (and avoid milkshakes!), you will eat only about 1100-1200 calories, depending on the food you eat. Lap-Band patients on average lose about 1.5-2 pounds a week.

But a good patient in a good program with education and exercise can lose 2-3 pounds per week. I know because I have seen it happen in my own clinic! You'll be able to eat most of the solid foods that you enjoy, just not as much of them as you used to.

Because you cannot eat very much food, it is important to focus on the most nutritious food. You will not have much room in your pouch to fill, so fill it with the most nutrition that you can. Remember, the Lap-Band does not affect your intestines to instigate malabsorption of fat, so you will need to make the right choices. So, not only does a good understanding of nutrition help with weight loss, it also helps with your overall health.

Potential problems and how to solve them

Some patients may have a little trouble with certain foods after the Lap-Band surgery, but this is not predictable. Some people have trouble with thick breads or biscuits, while others have no trouble with anything. A lot of this depends on your adjustments. If you just had an adjustment and your band is tight, you might be on liquids for a few days and work your way up to fish and chicken. It is important for you to be educated on all this, so that you know what to expect and can plan the timing of your adjustments around other events in your life.

If you are planning a cruise, do not get an adjustment right before you leave. Enjoy your cruise and when you return you can have your band adjusted. This is life! Some patients will fib to their doctors, saying they are too tight and need some fluid taken out of their band, and the doctor will later discover that they wanted to be able to eat a lot on their vacations! A good clinic will recognize that life has certain ups and downs that will affect your adjustment schedule. My goal is for my patients to have a good relationship with food so that they are able to enjoy vacation meals without overeating and putting weight back on.

There are complications with any surgery. Remember that the gastric bypass surgery has an average death rate of one to two percent, though one Medicare study found a 5% death rate. That means one patient in 20 died! With the Lap-Band, the mortality rate is .1% - that is one patient out of 1000 died. These are much better statistics. One of the most common surgeries is gall bladder removal. The death rate for that surgery is about 1 in 750 patients. The Lap-Band is even safer than this routine surgery. While the risks of any surgery must be considered, they are very low for the Lap-Band. The American Institute of Gastric Banding (AIGB) is a group of surgery centers and doctors around the U.S. They have the largest collection of Lap-Band numbers. As a group, they have done more than 10,000 Lap-Bands and have had zero deaths.

Other risks of the Lap-Band surgery are:

- Deep vein thrombosis, or blood clots in the legs that could travel to the lungs. If it is not detected, it can cause death. A good Lap-Band surgeon will have a whole program built around this possibility: leg squeezers during and after surgery, blood thinners around the time of surgery, and sometimes blood thinners after the surgery if the patient is at high risk of developing clots. The staff should know that if you call and say your right leg is swollen to twice the size of your left leg, it is a serious condition requiring immediate hospitalization. Fortunately, I have not encountered this problem and it is quite rare. However, if you or a loved one is considering having Lap-Band surgery, you should check that there are procedures in place to minimize the risk of clot formation.

- Slippage. This is when your stomach slips around the Band, which is not a serious emergency. The old slippage rate was around 7%. With the new band introduced in 2007 and the new placement of the band, the rate is 3-4%. Slippage is most often caused by vomiting, so we try to ensure you are not vomiting around the time of surgery. The surgeon will prepare you before surgery by putting an anti-nausea patch behind your ear and instructing the anesthesiologist not to give medicines that can cause nausea. The recovery nurse knows to evaluate any stomach problems you may feel after surgery. If you do experience slippage, you might need to go to the hospital and have the surgery redone.

- Erosion. On the internet you might find articles along the lines of "My Lap-Band Ate Through My Stomach." With the old Band, surgeons used to do more dissection around the stomach, which might cause a little hole in the back of the stomach that over time would erode through. But erosion is very rare with the new way we do the surgery. If it does happen, we would just take the Lap-Band out. If there were a hole we would fix it, but usually your stomach would seal up by itself. After a couple of months, you could have the Lap-Band put back in.

- Problems with the port. The most common complication of the Lap-Band surgery involves the tubing and the port and is simple and fast to rectify. The port can (on rare occasions) flip, and the tubing can crack. The makers of the Lap-Band changed the design in response to these problems and reduced tubing complications from about 10% to about 5%. This type of problem can usually be corrected with a simple, outpatient day-surgery procedure through the same small incision of your original surgery.

- Nutritional deficiency. It is possible to have vitamin deficiency because old habits are hard to break and there is not much nutrition in chips and junk food. I always recommend that my patients take a multivitamin every day, at least for the first year after Lap-Band surgery. Meanwhile, I require that they attend support groups that teach about nutrition. I do not expect someone to suddenly eat a perfect diet after the surgery, but I do expect my patients to slowly adopt healthier eating patterns and focus on nutritious food. Since the procedure leaves space to consume only about 1100-1200 calories per day, those calories should be packed with good vitamins and minerals.

- Pregnancy. As women lose weight, their hormones become more regular and it is easier for them to get pregnant. I recommend taking some sort of birth control for two years after the surgery if you want to become pregnant (and obviously for longer if you wish to avoid pregnancy), so that you will be at a healthy weight starting out your pregnancy. If you do become pregnant, your surgeon can take all the fluid out of your band so it is like you never had the surgery. You can put on weight and have a healthy pregnancy, then fill the band back up after the pregnancy and you are done breastfeeding.

A study compared non-surgery patients, Lap-Band patients, and gastric bypass patients who were pregnant. It found that the non-surgery patients and the Lap-Band patients had on average the same size babies. The gastric bypass patients typically had smaller babies, which is not good since birth weight is very important to a baby's health. Most doctors consider a pregnant woman who has had gastric bypass to be high risk and will send her to a medical center for careful monitoring. If it were my family member looking to get pregnant, I would consider the Lap-Band as the only surgical weight-loss option.

- Putting weight back on. In this case, the patient should go back to the clinic. The surgeon will ascertain if there might be slippage or leakage of the band. Most of the time there is nothing wrong with the band and the weight gain is due to poor eating habits. This is possible if you tend to eat during times of stress and go through a tough time at work, or if you eat when you are depressed and go through a break-up. When you feel vulnerable, you are more likely to return to old habits. This is when a support group can be very helpful, even years after your surgery.

Complication rates

Dr. Ponce in Atlanta studied 1014 of his own Lap-Band cases and followed them for up to 4 years. The complications he found are very low. Out of 1014 cases, there were only 2 erosions and 5 tubing breaks, and only 8 bands were explanted (removed). No deaths occurred.

On average he had a 65% plus or minus 19% excess weight loss after four years. This means that while the average weight loss of his patients was 65% of their excess weight, some patients lost 84% of their excess weight, while some only lost 46%.

These different results came from the same surgeon and the same surgery. It is therefore the patient who is the variable. Because the Lap-Band is a straightforward surgery, it does not matter if you find the greatest surgeon to perform it. It is much more important to be a great patient – to be honest, to come back for follow-ups, to educate yourself on nutrition, and to attend support groups.

Lap-Band Percent Excess Weight Loss

%EWL

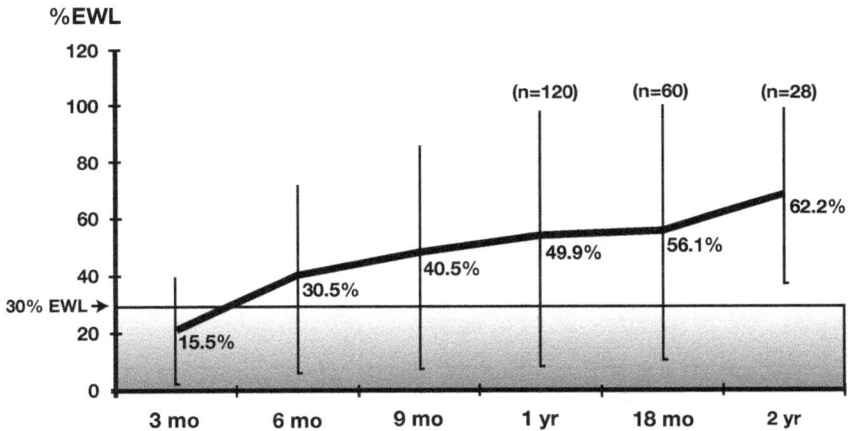

While the average weight-loss for Dr Ponce's patients after two years (and his rates are fairly typical) is about 62% of excess weight, patients who remain highly motivated, adopt a regular exercise plan that they enjoy (no, exercise need not be a grueling chore!), and continue to learn about nutrition and adapt their food choices accordingly can expect to lose nearly all of their excess weight. This is why I like to think of the Lap-Band as a tool, not as a solution in and of itself. Success ultimately depends on the individual patient's approach to using this tool.

Long-term Effectiveness

You may have heard some people say that you cannot have the Lap-Band if you have a lot of weight to lose. There are internet articles that claim that the Lap-Band is too conservative a procedure for losing a lot of weight and is only a bridge to the gastric bypass surgery. Just after the Lap-Band was approved, some doctors thought that way. Because it is an easy surgery, it can be safely performed on a high-risk patient, such as someone who weighs 600 pounds. So they thought that if they could perform this safe Lap-Band surgery, the patient might lose enough weight to be more stable and be able to undergo the gastric bypass. But as their heaviest of patients continued to lose weight with the Lap-Band, they found they did not need the gastric bypass at all. The patients were happy, lost the weight, and felt good.

This is a chart comparing the effectiveness of the old model of the Lap-Band (the solid line) and the gastric bypass (the dotted line) over the first 5 years after surgery.

5 Year Weight Loss Outcomes LAP-BAND vs, Gastric Bypass

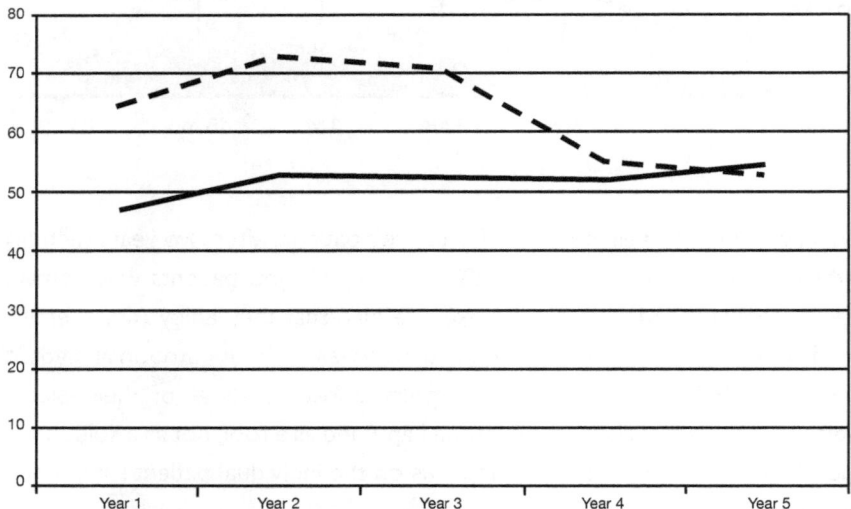

Gastric Bypass
LAP-BAND

FreemanJ., et al, Weight Loss After Extended Gastric Bypass, Obesity Surgery, 7, 1997, 337-344 O'Brien, et al, The Laprascopic Adjustable Gastric Band: A Prospective Study of Medium Term Effects of Weight, Health and QOL, Obesity Surgery, 12, 2002, 652-660

As we know from years of studies, the bypass works, and sometimes works too well. Patients their first year will lose on average 70% of their excess weight. But something happens around year three and they start to slowly put the weight back on. With the Lap-Band, patients do not lose weight as fast, maybe 40-45% of their excess weight during the first year. But they keep chugging along losing more. Five years down the road, the two lines meet. So why would a patient choose to have the surgery that requires stomach stapling and intestinal rerouting when he or she could have an outpatient surgery and go back to work in 3-5 days for the same long-term results? This chart indicates that while the gastric bypass is effective for losing weight, the Lap-Band is effective for losing weight *and* keeping it off.

With the new Lap-Band model, the results are even more impressive. The new band was approved in the United States in 2007, but they had it in Australia before. Dr. O'Brien's and Dr. Dixon's group in Australia compiled statistics on their patients who had the new version of the Lap-Band. They found that after one year the average excess weight lost by their patients was a little over 60%. So the difference in first year results between the new Lap-Band and the gastric bypass is much smaller than figure 18 indicates, because the new Lap-Band model is more effective. The lines will no longer take 5 years to meet; they will meet at 2-3 years. And after 5 years, the Lap-Banders will continue to lose excess weight, while the gastric bypass patients will, as we have seen, stay the same or possibly put weight back on.

As we saw above, the long-term benefits of losing weight are impressive. In January 2008, Dr. O'Brien and Dr. Dixon came out with a study that showed that 73% of their Lap-Band patients were cured of their diabetes. Their diabetes was not just treated with a pill, not better controlled, but *cured*. The patients are off their medicines and their hemoglobin A1c is normal. After they saw these results a couple of years ago, Dr. O'Brien has repeatedly said that if patients receive the Lap-Band within the first two years of their diagnosis with diabetes, almost all of them will be cured. But if they wait until they have had diabetes for ten years or more, most will be better controlled but almost no one will be cured of diabetes. That is because after so many years their pancreas gives out from working too hard. The statistics of cure rates among Lap-Band patients steadily decline between two and ten years.

I think that in the near future, when an overweight patient sees his or her primary care family doctor and is diagnosed with diabetes, the doctor will no longer recommend a diet plan as a first option, nor a shot or insulin treatment, but rather the Lap-Band surgery. The surgery is simply the most effective way to cure diabetes within two years of the diagnosis. If the patient and doctor wait and try other treatments first, it may be too late for the surgery to cure the disease.

Notes

Notes

Chapter Four
The Importance of a Program

Why do I need to follow a program after the surgery?

Part of why it's so hard for us to lose weight in this country is that companies like Nabisco, the makers of Oreo cookies, have to sell more cookies every year to make their stocks go up. A while ago Nabisco came up with Double Stuff Oreos that have twice the white filling. This worked out so well for their sales that they started making other Oreo products, like mini Oreo packs. The problem with these mini packs is most people eat three or four of them (and the same amount of cookie ends up costing more). People trying to lose weight tried Thinsation diet Oreos. To get kids more interested (as if kids don't gravitate towards Oreos on their own), the company came up with Oreo Barbi. There were commercials recently for Oreo pizzas and Cakesters. There are also fudge Oreos, mint Oreos, and orange Halloween Oreos. At the time I am writing this, there are 29 types of Oreo cookies. They taste good, are strategically placed in stores, seem pretty inexpensive, and infiltrate our television programs. It is very hard to resist Oreos, and this is just one of the many unhealthy products whose makers increase revenues by encouraging us to eat more than we should.

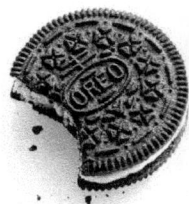

Oreo is a registered trademark of KF Holdings, Inc

Here is another quick quiz: which McDonald's item has the most calories — 4 hamburgers, a Big Mac, 2 sausage McGriddles, or a large chocolate shake?

Well, a Big Mac has 560 calories. Two sausage McGriddles have 840. Four hamburgers have 1040 calories. And a large chocolate shake has 1160! Most people do not expect the chocolate shake to be the highest in calories and think it is a fairly harmless post-meal treat. In actuality, it contains over half the calories nearly anyone should consume in a day. If you order a Big Mac, a large fries, a diet Coke, and a chocolate shake, that's 2100 calories for one pretty typical U.S. meal. This adds up to more calories than an average person needs in a whole day and is usually consumed in under 30 minutes. A good Lap-Band program can help educate patients about just these sorts of traps.

Food companies have to reveal this information on their web sites, so if you visit mcdonalds.com you can look up the calories for all the items. Also keep in mind that the high calories are only part of the problem – the meal described above is also an incredibly fatty meal and the food itself is of very low quality (even though it tastes good). McDonald's has to use really low quality meat in order to sell a burger for 99 cents and make enough money to pay their employees, cover their rent and other expenses, pay for all their advertising, and still turn a profit. The U.S. actually exports out most of the high quality meat the country produces precisely because of pressure from powerful companies who want the less expensive meats to remain in the U.S.

There are a lot of ways to take shortcuts and lose a few pounds rapidly, but do not underestimate how difficult it is to lose weight and keep it off in our country. Unhealthy eating habits have become routine in our country: children are served pizza and sodas at school, you will encounter hundreds of advertisements for fast and heavily processed food during the course of the day, and many of our friends, colleagues, and family members encourage us to indulge in calorie-dense foods in often unconscious ways. If you are reading this book, you are probably familiar with the difficulties any American trying to lose weight faces. A support group can help you combat all the tempting advertising for unhealthy foods, guide you through conflicting claims about weight-loss, provide you with effective strategies for recognizing and avoiding situations where you overeat, and educate you about nutrition.

What are some components I should look for in a program?

A good program should set you up with an introductory day where you meet with a dietician to help you be a smarter eater. You should have your weight and body measurements taken. You will also need to talk with the clinic's staff about your insurance coverage so they can help you with it (more on this tricky subject soon). They should guide you to informational reading materials on the Lap-Band, nutrition, and exercise. I cannot stress enough that the more you read, the better. You need to know where you are starting from to have reasonable expectations of where you want to get to. Ideally, this first clinic will also include a meeting with the surgeon who will perform your surgery. You should feel comfortable with the surgeon and feel that he or she understands you as an individual, not merely as another case.

A good program should have you meet with a dietician several times after the surgery to help you slowly reintroduce food into your system so that eventually you will be able to eat what you really enjoy. The dietician should talk with you about portion sizes, balanced meals, cooking strategies, and smart restaurant choices.

An effective program will set up regular meeting with you so you learn and stay motivated. I offer a special group called the perioperative support group, which is for people who are about to have or have just had the Lap-Band surgery. We cover six topics that are very important for patient success. Patients come to two groups before surgery and every week for four weeks after surgery. In addition, I require my patients to come to my clinic once per month for the first year after surgery. From the second year on, I like to see my patients every six months to make sure that they are doing well and that their bands are adjusted properly. There are many surgeons who do not see their patients until six weeks after surgery. That means the patient spends six weeks with this new band not knowing if they are eating the right things or eating too fast. Many clinics only want to see patients once a year or even every other year. This will not allow you to achieve your greatest weight-loss success and keep you happy. Regular clinic visits should be required.

There should be options for support groups that work with your schedule. Many programs only have support groups once a month. If you miss one because you do not feel well or get stuck in traffic, you would have to go two months on your own. My program offers group three times a week to ensure that everyone interested can attend on a very regular basis.

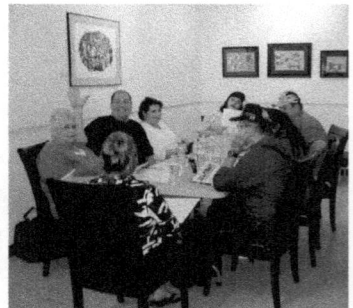

Support Group

Also, the doctor should lead many of the support groups, even though you should also be able to meet with nurses and dietitians. There are a lot of patients who only see their surgeon ten minutes before the surgery and never again. While nurses and dietitians can answer many questions, the surgeon should be available to address medical concerns. The surgeon should also understand what his or her patients experience so he or she can remain informed.

If you come to see your doctor every six months for the rest of your life, it is important that you like your surgeon and your clinic. Patients can choose their program, and programs should also be choosy in their patients. I have turned away patients that I knew were not a good fit for my program. You should not get the feeling that the clinic sees you as just a source of income – they should be genuinely interested in your long-term health. You, in turn, should feel like it is a place you would be happy to go to fairly frequently. If you have to drive a long ways, if you do not like the staff, if you are physically uncomfortable in the waiting room or offices, or if there is any other aspect of the program that you find unappealing, you should probably look into other options.

The program should have someone trained in insurance verification to see what your benefits really are. This person should know the right questions to ask the insurance company. If an individual calls their insurance company 100 different times, he or she might get 100 different answers, spend hours on the phone, and be turned down for Lap-Band coverage. If you know the specific codes and whom to talk with, you can get a straight answer and possibly better results.

The insurance company will require a lot of documentation, and a good clinic will help you track it down. You will have to show that you have been overweight for at least the last five years in a row, meaning you will have to submit notes from your doctor confirming that every year your BMI was over 40 or over 35 with comorbidities. Patients who are missing a note from one year are often denied. One patient I see in my support groups beat cancer and saw her doctor every month for chemotherapy, but she was too embarrassed to weigh in. So she has no documentation that she was overweight and was denied insurance coverage for Lap-Band surgery. (Please do not feel embarrassed about being weighed at the doctor's office; not only is it an important record for insurance purposes, it can also help you to understand what reasonable weight-loss goals for different time frames are. Doctors' scales are also usually a lot more accurate than scales bought for homes and do not read out five pounds lighter if you shake them, turn them to the left, and put your right foot in the air. More and more doctors also have scales that can accurately read weights up to 1000 pounds.) In addition, all insurance companies require you to see a psychologist or psychiatrist before they will approve your Lap-Band surgery. Other requirements vary by insurance company.

A program should offer loan options so that you can finance your surgery if you do not go through your insurance. There are companies like Care Credit and there are banks that will offer loans for surgeries. The amount you pay per month for 36 months will be about the same as what you will be saving on food and medicine. There are many factors that influence whether or not to have the surgery, but financing should not be one of them.

It is the responsibility of the clinic to educate patients before surgery and help prepare them for the surgery. A program should do an Optifast or similar meal-replacement program before the surgery, obtain your cardiac history, and perhaps even have you see a pulmonologist if you have sleep apnea. The surgery should be done as safely as possible, and you should feel confident that the clinic is doing everything it can to make your surgery safe.

The clinic should also help you decide when the best time is for a post-operative adjustment. It is not a good idea to adjust the band right before you go on vacation, to a wedding, or to a stressful family reunion. You should be able to handle these types of situations without struggling with a recently adjusted band. Enjoy the vacation, have fun at the wedding, tell your relatives how you feel, and come back later for your adjustment. You should observe how your eating patterns change in these contexts so that you can learn from your behaviors; adjusting the Lap-Band is not the best way to confront stress eating or other detrimental behaviors.

A program should be comprehensive and have your long-term goals in mind. It's easier for patients to stay on track if everyone they need to see – the surgeon, a dietician, a nurse, a psychiatrist, a pulmonologist, a cardiologist, etc. – is in one location. Nobody has time to travel around every week or month to see all these different people, which means that if this is the only option you will likely not see specialists as often as you should and your care will not be as good. Of course, you should be allowed to continue seeing your regular doctors, but there should be easy options for you to keep on top of your health.

A good program should also set up an individualized exercise regimen with a physical therapist. The therapist should be trained to work with people with joint problems and other health complications. You should learn about low-impact options at the beginning and be able to safely adjust the exercise program as you lose weight, have fewer health problems, and have more energy. You do not need to have an expensive gym membership to exercise. There are usually lower-cost options at community college facilities, the YMCA, local swimming pools, or community classes. A physical therapist could also show you exercises you can do in your home or around your neighborhood. If you want to use high-tech equipment, you can of course pay $50 a month for a gym membership, but this membership does not mean you will exercise more effectively than if you choose lower-cost options.

A good program should also help you make family adjustments and encourage you to work with your family and friends at weight loss. It is hard to maintain a healthy new lifestyle if you are surrounded with friends and family who offer you unhealthy foods and encourage you to watch a television show rather than go on a walk. The Lap-Band surgery will not only affect you; it will affect the dynamics of your relationships with other people.

What can I do to be a good patient?

The patient's responsibility is to learn and keep learning. You need to be willing to make a lifestyle change. Food is only one part of the equation; activity and exercise is the other part of it. If you continue to put yourself in the same situations with the same people, either you will not be successful or you will be unhappy. A good program should help you to be happy and not always worrying about your weight. The doctors should worry about your weight, and the patient should worry about making the right choices and being content with a healthy new lifestyle.

A patient has the responsibility to keep in touch. There are a lot of people who do want help, and the surgery clinic will eventually stop trying to encourage a reluctant patient to attend support groups or come in for check-ups. You should understand that with the Lap-Band, you are not just committing to a quick surgical procedure; you are committing to making a lifestyle change that will last for the remainder of your life.

The new changes you will be making in your life provide you with an exciting opportunity to give back to your community. I have partnered my clinic with non-profit organizations that have active

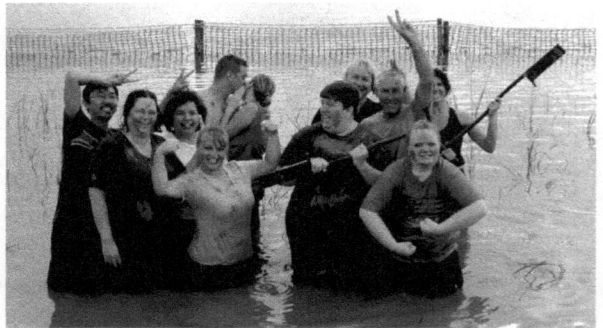

Grass Planting, Texas City Prairie Preserve

volunteering opportunities, which are a fun way to get exercise while doing something beneficial and often fun. My patients and my staff periodically plant marsh grasses around the Galveston Bay area to help rebuild the habitat and develop muscles with all the digging. I also find that focusing on community events helps people to step outside of themselves. It is so easy in our society to become isolated, which can lead to lots of television watching and mindless snacking. Connecting with others in meaningful ways ultimately helps with long-term weight loss and maintenance. There are also local walks that benefit various worthy causes, like breast cancer research, scholarship funds, leukemia treatments – you name it.

Most importantly, you need to be willing to fully acknowledge all aspects of your current lifestyle and be willing to change the unhealthy components of it. This can be very difficult, and your clinic should provide you with much support in different forms. For example, many parents say their children refuses to eat this or that healthy food. But children do not really have a choice. If you offer them healthy foods, they will either eat them or go hungry. A baby who is given broccoli, chicken, tofu, bell peppers, and other healthy foods will eat them and like them, usually for their whole life. A baby who is given cookies and fast food will eat those and like those for the rest of their lives. Patients who make poor food choices often need to relearn habits that were formed in early childhood, which cannot happen overnight. They need to be retrained on how to eat well, and that is why regular meetings with a dietician are so important.

Many patients of mine have said that they do not know why they are three hundred pounds because they never eat. I like to use a calorimeter machine, which you breathe into for about five minutes. It gives your resting metabolic rate, which is how many calories you would have to consume to maintain your current weight if all you did every day was lie in bed and breathe. Our average pre-Lap-Band patient blows about 2500 calories. This means that they are consuming more than 2500 calories per day, because they expend additional calories by doing housework, working, talking on the telephone, driving, and otherwise leading their lives. Even these minor activities burn more calories than lying in bed. You cannot get to where you want to be if you do not know where you are starting from. It is a harsh reality check for a lot of people to learn they are consuming 3000 or 4000 calories a day. As a good patient, you need to be ready to accept some difficult truths and take full responsibility for your health. A good clinic will be compassionate but will not accept excuses.

Notes

Notes

Chapter Five
Financial Considerations

How much does it cost?

It depends on whether or not you go through an insurance company. If you want to go through insurance, the first question is "Is it a covered benefit?" If it is not, the insurance will not pay for it no matter what. If it is a covered benefit, the next question is "What is my out-of-pocket amount?" You should expect to have to pay the whole out-of-pocket amount, typically $3000 or $5000, depending on your policy. Insurance will not cover any meal-replacement products or dietician visits, so this will be another expense on top of your out-of-pocket amount.

Most companies also require you to have participated in a doctor-monitored weight loss program for 4-6 months. Jenny Craig and Weight Watchers do not count, because they are not overseen by a doctor. If you do not have any record of participation in a qualified program, then this may be an additional expense, in terms of both money and time. So it can really take six months to a year for approval. My clinic averages about 7 months. That means that if you signed up for the program tomorrow and wanted to go through your insurance company, you would not have your surgery until about 7 months from now.

Many patients opt to avoid all this and pay cash. The cash prices vary – many are around $14,000 or $15,000. This sounds like a lot, but it is less than a Honda Civic, and you can probably find financing options that will let you pay it through installments. This price should include a comprehensive program and adjustments for the fist year. After that, most surgeons charge about $150 per adjustment, which you may need about once or twice a year.

Your life will change

Take a moment and think about what aspects of your life would improve if you lost extra weight and had better health.

I often hear the following concerns:

- My husband and I are about to retire and we want to travel. But my knees hurt, my back hurts, and it is hard to get around a cruise ship, especially those narrow stairs.

- I just had my first grandchild and I want to be around for her for a long time to watch her grow up.

- I cannot keep up with my kids anymore. I used to coach soccer and play softball with them, but now I just give them the ball and tell them to play outside. I feel like I'm missing out on important bonding experiences.

- My relationship with my spouse is not good because I don't feel good about myself.

- I would love to see my old high school friends again, but I'm not up to attending the reunion.

To me, time is the most important thing in the world. You will never get time back – you will miss more opportunities, more events, and more quality experiences with loved ones. Many people make a New Year's resolution to lose weight, start exercising, or become healthy. But then a year goes by, nothing has changed, and they make the same resolution. When it comes to weight loss, the longer you wait to make a change, the worse the problem gets.

It is not really a question of whether you can afford to join a program or get the surgery. It is really a question of whether you can afford NOT to do something about your weight. I encourage you to look into your covered insurance benefits and investigate financing options if you decide that you want the Lap-Band surgery but are concerned about paying for it.

Notes

Chapter Six
Patient profiles

Jim

Jim had the Lap-Band surgery at the end of February 2008. Here is his story as of August 2008.

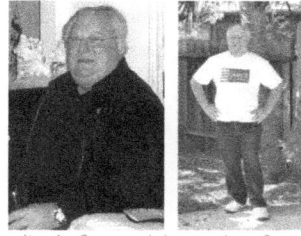

Jim before and 6 months after the Lap-Band

It has been a terrific ride for me.

Before I had the Lap-Band surgery, my health problems kept multiplying. First I had high blood pressure. Then I developed type 2 diabetes and was on three medications for it. I had severe obstructive sleep apnea and needed to use a sleep apnea machine to get rest at night. My knees were so bad I could not walk even to get around at work and in the house and I began taking cortisone shots. I took a stress test in January and the doctor said I was wearing my heart out and would have a severe problem very shortly if I did not do something about my weight. But it is hard to lose weight when you cannot exercise because you are too big! So my doctor highly recommended I look into the Lap-Band surgery.

On February 26, I had the surgery. Afterwards, I took a couple of days off work and relaxed a bit. Then I began to do a lot of walking. It was slow, because I was pretty big. In six months I lost 51 pounds, and now it is very easy for me to walk a couple of miles. I'm 63 years old and have a couple more years until retirement. I'm looking more forward to retirement now than I was six months ago, because I will be able to do so much more.

Medically, my Hemoglobin A1c, the average over a three-month period, is down to 5.2, which is normal. That means my blood sugars are between 90 and 100, which is normal, over a three-month period. I am not taking any medications for diabetes any more. I do not need the sleep apnea machine now, either. I do take a blood pressure medication still, but the doctor said as soon as I lose a few more pounds and break that 200-pound barrier I could probably stop it.

I joined a fitness center and started working out. I built up my strength and am now getting really into the exercise. This past Sunday I burned 1600 calories just walking. Six months ago I could not walk and thought exercise was a dirty word!

The Lap-Band may seem expensive at first, but I have found that I am quickly saving money by ceasing nearly all of my previous medications. I do not go out to eat as often as I used to, because there are other things I enjoy doing now. When I do go out to eat, the bill is much lower because I just order an appetizer or split an entrée with my wife. I used to eat everything on my plate and then half of what she was eating. I do not make trips to the grocery store as often as I used to, either. So pretty soon the Lap-Band will have paid for itself.

Since the Lap-Band surgery, I have never been sick, not even right after the surgery. Some people might feel nauseated afterwards, and your surgeon should give you a medication you can take if you need to.

I have a good social life. People at work are just amazed. When I see people now I have not seen in a while, they have to do a double-take. Even my regular doctor was surprised when I went for a check-up a few weeks ago – I was 212 at my weigh-in with him and he said it had been a long time since he saw me at that weight.

Group sessions are important to me. A lot of clinics just leave you on your own after the surgery. They do not have any follow up or group sessions. I look forward to the chance to talk with other people about what we are all experiencing, and I learn a lot from what others are doing. I still attend support group sessions at Dr. Vuong's clinic occasionally to keep myself motivated.

My one regret is that I did not get the Lap-Band sooner. I enjoy my life so much more now.

Sandra

Sandra has lost 100 pounds in the six months since her Lap-Band surgery.   Here is her story.

I've struggled with my weight for nearly 30 years. I've experienced high blood pressure, low energy, intense rheumatoid arthritis, and

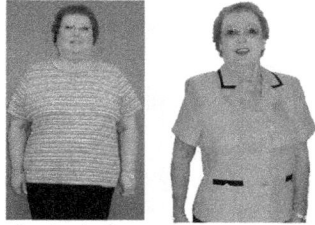

Sandra before and 6 months after the Lap-Band

sore legs and knees. I was perpetually tired and running low on confidence. Even something as simple as bending down would make me short of breath. And I got discouraged from trying different diets that never fit my lifestyle.

After both my doctor and my husband warned me of the serious health problems my weight would inevitably continue to cause, I began to research the possibility of surgery. I saw advertisements for Lap-Band surgeons, but my real encouragement came from a customer at the store where I work. She raved about the positive and rewarding outcomes she had experienced with the Lap-Band.

I then decided to go with my husband to meet with Dr. Vuong and learn more about the procedure. I attended an informational seminar that walked me through the surgery, life afterwards, and the costs. I decided this was the perfect option for me.

I went on a 1200-calorie regimen for a week before my surgery, which helped me get a sense of the healthier portions I would eat after getting the band. My husband went on the diet as well and has continued on it now that I have had my surgery. He has been very supportive and has ended up losing 40 pounds!

Just six months after my Lap-Band procedure, I've already lost 100 pounds! It's been almost 30 years since I was at this weight. My ultimate goal is to lose just 20 more pounds, and I know the support groups the clinic offers will help me. I still go regularly, about every two weeks.

There are things I can do now that I could not do before the surgery. My blood pressure has normalized, I no longer fight acid reflux, the aches in my legs and feet are gone, and my rheumatoid arthritis has abated. I feel better physically and I am a happier, more content person.

Notes

Chapter Seven
Some common questions

Q: Why are the insurance companies not getting on board with the Lap-Band surgery? Why is it so difficult to get them to cover it?

A: Insurance companies train their employees to look for every way possible to deny coverage. Their goal is to spend as little money as possible, and they look into this not from a long-term perspective, but from a day-to-day perspective. If they approved the Lap-Band surgery for a patient, they would ultimately spend less on covering medications and doctor's visits over a number of years. But on one specific day, it is less expensive for them to cover a few prescription refills than a surgery. The system is broken and backwards.

Q: How long do you stay in the surgery center during the surgery?

A: Most people who come in at 6 or 8 in the morning will be home by 1 or 1:30PM. The surgery itself only takes about 30 minutes, but the clinic will need some time to prepare you and will want to monitor you for a while afterwards.

Q: What can I do to lose the most weight?

A: Understand that it is a process. You won't wake up skinny or knowing all the answers. It is a partnership between the patient and the program. You have to love your clinic and your surgeon and be willing to visit them often, be honest with them, and be willing to make some significant changes in many aspects of your life.

Q: Can I join another program if I already had the Lap-Band surgery?

A: There is an unwritten rule in this field that no surgeon will touch another surgeon's Lap-Band. That is because if the surgeon does the Lap-Band surgery, and another surgeon does an adjustment, the second surgeon will take on the responsibility for all the risks and complications that may have resulted from the initial surgery. It sounds rather self-serving, but remember that surgeons have very hefty insurance fees and requirements as well, so they do not want to take on unnecessary risks. Sometimes there are exceptions, but it is important to find a surgeon and program you are comfortable with before you have the surgery. Do some research, attend some seminars, and find the best fit for you.

Q: Can I have the surgery done in Mexico to save some money?

If you go to Mexico for the surgery, there is hardly any surgeon in the United States who will touch it. You would have to travel back to Mexico for your adjustments, which would end up costing you more in the long-run. Also, consistent follow-up and support is the most important element for weight-loss success. So unless you are willing to make regular trips to Mexico, this is highly unadvisable.

Q: How long will I need to take off work after the surgery?

A: Most people are back to work in three to five days, depending on their job. A few people with desk jobs even go back the next day, though I advise against that.

Q: Is there an age limit for the surgery?

A: The Medicare recommendation is 71. It depends, though. There are some 60-year-olds who are very old, and operating on them would be risky, and there are some 72-year-olds who are young and active, who would be good candidates for surgery. So it really depends on the patient's overall health.

Currently the Lap-Band is FDA approved only for patients over 18 years old, but I think that recommendation will change around spring 2009, when newer research will be released that shows the Lap-Band is an effective surgery in adolescents.

No matter your age, ask your surgeon if the Lap-Band surgery is right for you.

Q: If you have a problem with your gall bladder, can you have it removed at the same time as you have the Lap-Band surgery?

A: While it is possible to remove your gallbladder at the same time, most surgeons generally will not remove the gall bladder because there is bacteria inside it. Because the band is a foreign material being introduced into your body, the internal environment should remain as sterile as possible to reduce risks of infection or other complications.

Q: Where do you have adjustments done?

A: Usually they are done in the surgeon's office and only take a few minutes.

About the Author

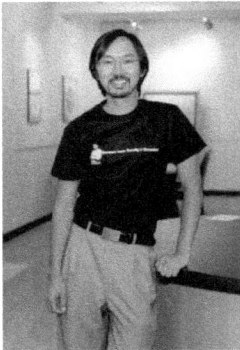

Dr. Vuong is a renowned Lap-Band surgeon from the Houston area. He received his education at Rice University, Texas A&M Medical School, completed surgical residency at St. Joseph's Hospital in Houston and currently practices in the Houston and Clear Lake areas. He is nationally recognized for his development of a successful support group program (available to patients in person and via DVD) that keeps patients on track for their long-term weight loss goals. Dr. Vuong believes that preoperative education and postoperative support groups are the key to becoming a happy, successful gastric band patient. He lives in the Houston area with his long time partner Melissa and their 2 year old daughter, Kizzie. To learn more about Dr. Vuong please visit www.TexasCitySurgical.com and www.MoreFromMyBand.com.

Dr. Vuong also believes in giving to charity, not only as a personal philosophy, but also a necessity for long term weight maintenance. His clinic and patients regularly participate in various fund-raiser walks and social community activities, like beach clean-ups. In addition, a portion of every cash lap-band surgery is also donated to the Snowdrop Foundation in that patient's name. Snowdrop Foundation in a nonprofit organization that raises money to provide scholarships for college tuition to survivors of childhood cancer.

Dr. Vuong also awards free lap-band surgeries to patients who have demonstrated significant charitable giving. To find out more about this program, please visit www.MoreFromMyBand.com

www.ingramcontent.com/pod-product-compliance
Lightning Source LLC
Chambersburg PA
CBHW030029290326
41934CB00005B/544